Superfoods or Super Toxins: How Oxalates Can Harm Your Health and What You Can Do About It

Judy kelly

Copyright © 2023, Judy Kelly.

All rights reserved. No part of this book may be reproduced or transmitted in any form or by any means, electronic or mechanical, including photocopying, recording, or by any information storage and retrieval system, without the written permission of the author.

Table of content

Chapter 1
Introduction
- Overview of Oxalates
- Importance of Understanding Oxalates in Our Diet
- Sources of Oxalates in Food
- Role of Oxalates in the Body

Chapter 2
- Health Conditions Linked to High Oxalate Levels
- Diagnosis and Testing for Oxalate Sensitivity
- Lists of High and Low Oxalate Foods

Chapter 3
- Managing Oxalate-Associated Health Conditions
- Treatment and Management of High Oxalate Levels

Conclusion
- Summary of Key Points
- Future Research Directions
- Resources for Further Information

Chapter 1

Introduction

Overview of Oxalates

Oxalates are naturally occurring substances found in many foods, including fruits, vegetables, nuts, and grains. They are also produced by the body as a byproduct of metabolism. While oxalates are essential for certain bodily functions, high levels of oxalates in the diet or the body can cause harm to our health. In this essay, we will discuss what oxalates are, their sources, their role in the body, and their potential dangers.

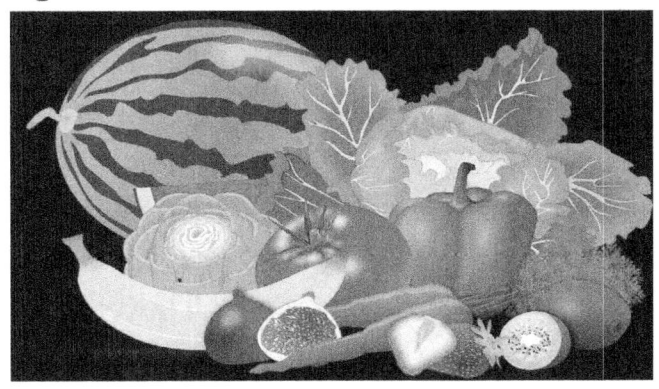

Oxalates, also known as oxalic acid, are a type of organic acid that can bind with minerals such as calcium to form crystals. These crystals can accumulate in various parts of the body, such as the kidneys, and lead to the formation of kidney stones. Oxalates are also found in many plant-based foods, including spinach, rhubarb, beet greens, nuts, and chocolate. They are also found in some fruits, such as berries, and some grains such as wheat bran, and are also produced by the body as a byproduct of metabolism.

In terms of chemical structure, oxalates are made up of two carbon atoms and two oxygen atoms, and they can exist in both the free form (oxalic acid) and the bound form (oxalates). They can be found in many plant-based foods and are especially concentrated in spinach, rhubarb, beet greens, nuts, and chocolate. They are also found in some fruits, such as berries, and some grains such as wheat bran. Oxalates are also produced by the body as a byproduct of metabolism, specifically when the body breaks down certain amino acids (glycine, hydroxyproline) and vitamin C.

In terms of their effect on the body, oxalates can be beneficial in small amounts as they play a role in the formation of bones and teeth, and the regulation of blood sugar levels. However, when the levels of oxalates in the body become too high, they can cause harm. High levels of oxalates can lead to the formation of kidney stones and can also contribute to the development of autoimmune diseases, neurological symptoms, and gastrointestinal symptoms.

It's important to note that when it comes to oxalates, the levels in food can vary greatly depending on the way it is grown and prepared, so it's essential to be aware of the potential dangers of high oxalate intake and to take steps to manage our intake of oxalates to reduce the risk of harm.

The human body needs a certain amount of oxalates for normal bodily functions. For example, oxalates play a role in the formation of bones and teeth, and the regulation of blood sugar levels. However, when the levels of oxalates in the body become too high, they can cause harm. High levels of oxalates can lead to the formation of kidney stones and can also contribute to the development of autoimmune diseases, neurological symptoms, and gastrointestinal symptoms.

One of the main dangers of high oxalate intake is the formation of kidney stones. Kidney stones are formed when oxalates bind with calcium in the urine to form crystals. These crystals can then accumulate in the kidneys and form stones. High oxalate intake can also contribute to the development of autoimmune diseases, such as rheumatoid arthritis and lupus, as well as neurological symptoms such as neuropathy and seizures, and gastrointestinal symptoms such as abdominal pain and diarrhea.

To reduce the risk of harm from high oxalate intake, it is important to identify high oxalate foods and to manage our intake of these foods. Testing for oxalates in food is one way to identify high oxalate foods, and there are also lists of high and low oxalate foods available. Strategies for lowering oxalate intake include avoiding high oxalate foods and consuming low oxalate foods, as well as managing any underlying health conditions that may contribute to high oxalate levels in the body.

In conclusion, oxalates are naturally occurring substances found in many foods, and they play a role in many normal bodily functions. However, high levels of oxalates in the diet or the body can cause harm to our health. It is important to be aware of the potential dangers of high oxalate intake and to take steps to manage our intake of oxalates to reduce the risk of harm. This can include identifying high oxalate foods, avoiding them and consuming low oxalate foods, and managing any underlying health conditions that may contribute to high oxalate levels in the body.

Importance of Understanding Oxalates in Our Diet

Understanding the role of oxalates in our diet is important for maintaining good health and preventing the development of certain health conditions. Oxalates, also known as oxalic acid, are a type of organic acid that can bind with minerals such as calcium to form crystals. These crystals can accumulate in various parts of the body, such as the kidneys, and lead to the formation of kidney stones. High levels of oxalates can also contribute to the development of autoimmune diseases, neurological symptoms, and gastrointestinal symptoms.

One of the main reasons to understand oxalates in our diet is to prevent the formation of kidney stones. Kidney stones are a common health problem and can cause severe pain, as well as other complications such as infections and blockages in the urinary tract. By understanding which foods are high in oxalates and limiting our intake of these foods, we can reduce our risk of developing kidney stones.

Another important reason to understand oxalates in our diet is to manage autoimmune diseases. Autoimmune diseases such as rheumatoid arthritis and lupus can be triggered or exacerbated by high levels of oxalates in the body. By managing our intake of oxalates, we can help reduce inflammation and symptoms associated with these conditions.

Moreover, understanding oxalates in our diet are important for managing neurological symptoms such as neuropathy and seizures, as well as gastrointestinal symptoms such as abdominal pain and diarrhea. High oxalate intake can contribute to these symptoms and by managing our intake of oxalates, we can help reduce their severity and frequency.

In addition, understanding oxalates in our diet can also help people who are on a special diet for medical reasons such as those with certain genetic conditions or those who have had organ transplants. For these people, high oxalate intake can cause serious health problems and they need to be aware of which foods are high in oxalates and manage their intake accordingly.

In conclusion, understanding the role of oxalates in our diet is important for maintaining good health and preventing the development of certain health conditions.

By understanding which foods are high in oxalates and limiting our intake of these foods, we can reduce our risk of developing kidney stones, autoimmune diseases, neurological symptoms, and gastrointestinal symptoms. It is important to be aware of the potential dangers of high oxalate intake and to take steps to manage our intake of oxalates to reduce the risk of harm.

Sources of Oxalates in Food

Oxalates are found in many foods, including fruits, vegetables, nuts, and grains. Some of the most common sources of oxalates in food include:

Spinach: Spinach is one of the highest oxalate-containing foods, with a high concentration of oxalates in the leaves.

Rhubarb: Rhubarb is another high oxalate food, with oxalates concentrated in the stalks.

Beet greens: Beet greens are also a high oxalate food, with oxalates concentrated in the leaves.

Nuts: Nuts such as almonds, cashews, and peanuts are high in oxalates.

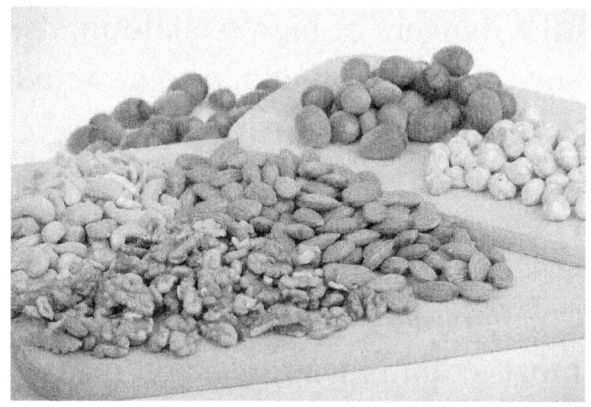

Chocolate: Chocolate is high in oxalates, especially dark chocolate.

Fruits: Some fruits such as berries (blackberries, raspberries, strawberries) and fruits with seeds or pits (such as plums, apricots, and kiwi) have moderate to high levels of oxalates.

Grains: Grains such as wheat bran, quinoa, and amaranth also have moderate to high levels of oxalates.

Legumes: Some legumes such as soybeans, black beans, navy beans, and kidney beans also contain moderate to high levels of oxalates.

Beverages: Some beverages such as tea and coffee are also sources of oxalates.

It's worth noting that the oxalate content of food can vary depending on how it is grown, prepared, and cooked. For example, boiling foods high in oxalates can reduce their oxalate content by up to 50%.

It's important to be aware of these food sources of oxalates and to manage our intake of these foods to reduce the risk of harm. Consulting with a dietitian or a healthcare professional can help identify oxalate foods and create a personalized diet plan that works for you.

It's also important to note that people who have a genetic condition called primary hyperoxaluria, which causes the body to produce excessive amounts of oxalates, may need to follow a low-oxalate diet and may need to avoid even moderate levels of oxalates in their food.

Role of Oxalates in the Body
Oxalates, also known as oxalic acid, play several roles in the body, some of which are beneficial while others can be harmful.

Formation of bones and teeth: Oxalates are necessary for the formation of bones and teeth. They bind with calcium to form crystals, which is an important component of bone and teeth formation.

Regulation of blood sugar levels: Oxalates play a role in regulating blood sugar levels by helping the body to absorb and utilize glucose.

Antioxidant properties: Oxalates have antioxidant properties and can help protect the body against cellular damage.

Formation of kidney stones: High levels of oxalates in the body can lead to the formation of kidney stones. Oxalates bind with calcium in the urine to form crystals, which can accumulate in the kidneys and form stones.

Autoimmune diseases: High levels of oxalates can contribute to the development of autoimmune diseases such as rheumatoid arthritis and lupus.

Neurological symptoms: High oxalate intake can contribute to the development of neurological symptoms such as neuropathy and seizures.

Gastrointestinal symptoms: High oxalate intake can also contribute to the development of gastrointestinal symptoms such as abdominal pain and diarrhea.

Detoxification: Oxalates can help the body detoxify by binding to toxins and heavy metals and helping to remove them from the body.

Inhibiting the growth of harmful microorganisms: Oxalates have antimicrobial properties and can inhibit the growth of harmful microorganisms, such as bacteria and fungi.

Interaction with Vitamin C: Oxalates can interfere with the absorption and utilization of vitamin C in the body when consumed in large amounts.

Interaction with calcium: High oxalate intake can also interfere with calcium absorption and metabolism in the body, which can lead to a risk of osteoporosis.

It's important to note that oxalates are essential for certain bodily functions, but high levels of oxalates in the body can cause harm. Therefore, it's important to be aware of the potential dangers of high oxalate intake and to take steps to manage our intake of oxalates to reduce the risk of harm.

It's also important to note that the effects of oxalates on the body can vary depending on the individual, as well as other factors such as overall health status, diet, and underlying medical conditions.

Chapter 2.

Health Conditions Linked to High Oxalate Levels

1. **Kidney Stones**
One of the main dangers of high oxalate intake is the formation of kidney stones. Kidney stones are formed when oxalates bind with calcium in the urine to form crystals. These crystals can then accumulate in the kidneys and form stones.

Kidney stones can cause severe pain and discomfort, and they can also lead to other complications such as infections and blockages in the urinary tract. If a kidney stone becomes stuck in the urinary tract, it can block the flow of urine and cause severe pain, nausea, and vomiting. In some cases, kidney stones can also cause bleeding and infection. If the stone is too large to pass through the urinary tract, surgery may be necessary to remove it.

The risk of developing kidney stones is increased by high levels of oxalates in the diet, as well as other factors such as low fluid intake, high intake of animal protein, and certain medical conditions such as gout and inflammatory bowel disease. People who have a history of kidney stones or a family history of kidney stones are also at an increased risk.

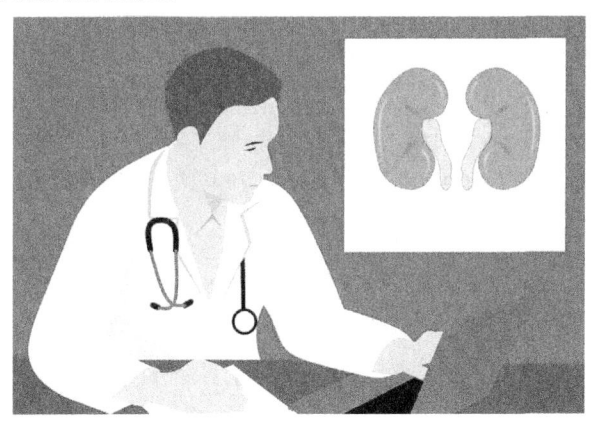

To reduce the risk of kidney stones, it's important to manage our intake of oxalates by avoiding high-oxalate foods and consuming low-oxalate foods. It's also important to drink plenty of water to help flush out the kidneys and reduce the formation of crystals.

2. **Autoimmune Disease**

Another danger of high oxalate intake is its potential contribution to the development of autoimmune diseases. Autoimmune diseases occur when the immune system mistakenly attacks healthy cells and tissues in the body. High levels of oxalates in the body can contribute to the development of autoimmune diseases such as rheumatoid arthritis and lupus by increasing inflammation and damaging healthy cells and tissues.

Rheumatoid arthritis is an autoimmune disease that causes inflammation and damage to the joints and other parts of the body. Lupus is a chronic autoimmune disease that can affect the skin, joints, kidneys, and other organs. High levels of oxalates can contribute to the development of these diseases by increasing inflammation and exacerbating symptoms.

High oxalate intake can also contribute to other autoimmune diseases such as Hashimoto's thyroiditis, Scleroderma, and fibromyalgia.

The exact link between oxalates and autoimmune diseases is not fully understood, but research suggests that high levels of oxalates in the body can activate the immune system and increase inflammation, leading to autoimmune diseases.

It's important to note that the development of autoimmune diseases is influenced by multiple factors, including genetics, environment, and lifestyle. Therefore, managing our intake of oxalates is just one step in reducing the risk of autoimmune diseases.

3. **Neurological symptoms**: High oxalate intake can contribute to the development of neurological symptoms such as neuropathy (nerve damage) and seizures. Research suggests that high levels of oxalates can damage nerve cells and disrupt nerve function, leading to neurological symptoms.

4. **Gastrointestinal symptoms**: High oxalate intake can also contribute to the development of gastrointestinal symptoms such as abdominal pain, diarrhea, and constipation. Oxalates can irritate the gut lining and cause inflammation, leading to these symptoms. They can also bind with calcium in the gut and form crystals, which can cause blockages and obstructions in the gastrointestinal tract.

It's important to note that the development of neurological and gastrointestinal symptoms is influenced by multiple factors, including genetics, environment, and lifestyle. Therefore, managing our intake of oxalates is just one step in reducing the risk of these symptoms.

5. **Autism**: Autism Spectrum Disorder (ASD) is a neurodevelopmental disorder characterized by difficulties with social interaction, communication, and repetitive behaviors. The exact cause of autism is not well understood, but it is thought to be related to a combination of genetic and environmental factors.

There is some evidence to suggest that high levels of oxalates in the body may contribute to the development of autism symptoms. Studies have found that children with autism have higher levels of oxalates in their urine compared to typically developing children.

Research suggests that people with autism may have an abnormal sensitivity to certain chemicals and substances in the body, including oxalates. Some studies have found that a low oxalate diet may improve symptoms of autism, such as hyperactivity, irritability, and repetitive behaviors.

It is important to note that autism is a complex and multidimensional condition and that a low oxalate diet may help some people but not others. A proper diagnosis and treatment plan should be done by a healthcare professional.

It is important to note that the relationship between oxalates and autism is still in the early stage of research and more studies are needed to confirm the correlation.

6. **Depression**: Depression is a mental disorder characterized by persistent feelings of sadness, hopelessness, and loss of interest in activities. It can also cause physical symptoms such as changes in appetite and sleep patterns, fatigue, and difficulty concentrating. The exact causes of depression are not well understood, but it is

thought to be related to a combination of genetic, environmental, and psychological factors.

There is some evidence to suggest that high levels of oxalates in the body may contribute to the development of depression. Studies have found that people with depression have higher levels of oxalates in their urine compared to healthy controls.

It is also known that some foods that are high in oxalates, such as spinach and beet greens, are also high in folate, which is a B vitamin that plays a role in mood regulation.

It is important to note that depression is a complex and multidimensional condition and that a low oxalate diet may help some people but not others. A proper diagnosis and treatment plan should be done by a healthcare professional.

It is important to note that the relationship between oxalates and depression is still in early research and more studies are needed to confirm the correlation.

Diagnosis and Testing for Oxalate Sensitivity

1. Urine oxalate testing

Urine oxalate testing is a way to measure the level of oxalates in the body. It involves collecting a urine sample and measuring the number of oxalates present. This test can help determine if a person has high levels of oxalates in their body, which may indicate an increased risk for certain health conditions such as kidney stones or fibromyalgia.

The test is usually done by a healthcare professional and it is a non-invasive test that can be done in a clinic or at home using a test kit.

It's important to note that a high level of oxalates in the urine doesn't necessarily mean that a person has an oxalate sensitivity or that they will develop related health conditions, but it can be an indication that a person may have a higher risk of developing these conditions and it can be used as a marker to monitor the effect of a low oxalate diet or other interventions.

It's also important to note that urine oxalate testing may not be covered by insurance and that it is not a routine test, so it may require a referral from a healthcare professional.

2. **Genetic testing**

Genetic testing is a way to analyze a person's DNA to identify variations or mutations that may increase their risk for certain health conditions or diseases. Genetic testing can help identify inherited genetic factors that may contribute to the development of certain health conditions that are associated with high oxalate levels such as kidney stones, fibromyalgia, and autism.

Several genetic tests can be done to identify variations in genes that may affect the metabolism of oxalates in the body. For example, genetic testing can identify variations in genes that are involved in the metabolism of Vitamin B6, which plays a role in the metabolism of oxalates.

It's important to note that genetic testing is not a routine test and it is not necessary for everyone, it is usually recommended for people who have a family history of certain health conditions associated with high oxalate levels, or for people who have been diagnosed with these conditions.

It's also important to note that genetic testing may not be covered by insurance and that it should be done by a licensed healthcare professional that can interpret the results and provide the appropriate counseling.

It's also important to note that the relationship between genetic testing and high oxalate levels is still in the early stage of research and more studies are needed to confirm the correlation.

3. **Laboratory testing:** One of the most accurate methods of identifying high-oxalate foods is laboratory testing. This can be done by sending samples of food to a laboratory for analysis. The laboratory will measure the number of oxalates in the food and provide a report of the results. This method is generally used for research purposes or for testing large batches of food.

4. **Food databases**: Several food databases list the oxalate content of different foods. These databases can

be accessed online and can be a useful tool for identifying high-oxalate foods. However, it's important to note that the oxalate content of food can vary depending on how it is grown, prepared, and cooked, so it's important to use these databases as a guide rather than a definitive answer.

5. **Consulting a dietitian or healthcare professional**: Consulting a dietitian or healthcare professional can help identify high-oxalate foods. They can provide personalized advice based on an individual's health status, dietary needs, and medical history.

6. **Testing at home**: There are some home testing kits available that allow you to test the oxalate content of food at home, these kits can be a good option for people who want to test a small number of foods.

It's important to note that the results of laboratory testing, food databases, and home testing kits may not be entirely accurate and may vary depending on the methods used. Therefore, it's important to consult with a dietitian or healthcare professional to get a more accurate assessment of the oxalate content of food.

Additionally, cooking and preparation methods can also affect the oxalate content of foods. For example, boiling foods high in oxalates can reduce their oxalate content by up to 50%. Therefore, it's important to be aware of how the food is prepared and cooked when assessing its oxalate content.

It's also worth noting that some individuals may be more sensitive to oxalates than others, for example, people who have a genetic condition called primary hyperoxaluria, which causes the body to produce excessive amounts of oxalates, may need to follow a low-oxalate diet and may need to avoid even moderate levels of oxalates in their food.

Lists of High and Low Oxalate Foods
Another way to identify high and low oxalate foods is by using lists of high and low oxalate foods. These lists can be found online, in books, or by consulting a dietitian or healthcare professional.

High oxalate foods typically include:
- Spinach
- Rhubarb
- Beet greens
- Nuts (such as almonds, hazelnuts, and peanuts)
- Chocolate
- Berries (such as blackberries, raspberries, and strawberries)
- Wheat bran
- Quinoa
- Amaranth
- Soybeans

- Black beans
- Navy beans
- Kidney beans
- Tea and coffee

Low oxalate foods typically include:
- Meat and fish
- Dairy products
- Eggs
- Fruits (such as apples, bananas, and oranges)
- Vegetables (such as cauliflower, cucumbers, and lettuce)
- Grains (such as rice, oats, and barley)
- Legumes (such as lentils, peas, and pinto beans)

It's important to note that the oxalate content of food can vary depending on how it is grown, prepared, and cooked, so it's important to use these lists as a guide rather than a definitive answer. Additionally, it's important to consult with a healthcare professional to get a more accurate assessment of the oxalate content of food, particularly if you have a condition that makes you more sensitive to oxalates.

It's also important to keep in mind that everyone's dietary needs and sensitivities are different and that what might be a high-oxalate food for one person may not be for another. Additionally, some people may need to follow a low-oxalate diet to manage certain health conditions, such as kidney stones or primary hyperoxaluria. In these cases, it's essential to work with a healthcare professional to create a personalized diet plan that works for you.

It's also worth noting that just because a food is low in oxalates, it does not mean it's necessarily healthy. It's important to consider overall nutrient density and balance when incorporating low-oxalate foods into your diet.

Strategies for Lowering Oxalate Intake

There are several strategies for lowering oxalate intake and reducing the risk of harm:

Avoiding high oxalate foods: One of the most effective ways to lower oxalate intake is to avoid high oxalate foods. This can be done by using lists of high and low oxalate foods as a guide and consulting with a healthcare professional to get a more accurate assessment of the oxalate content of food.

Limiting portion sizes of high oxalate foods: Even if you can't avoid high oxalate foods entirely, you can still lower your oxalate intake by limiting portion sizes. Eating smaller amounts of high-oxalate foods can help reduce the overall amount of oxalates you consume.

Drinking plenty of water: Drinking plenty of water can help flush out the kidneys and reduce the formation of crystals, which can lead to kidney stones. Aim for at least eight glasses of water a day.

Cooking and preparation methods: Cooking and preparation methods can also affect the oxalate content of foods. For example, boiling foods high in oxalates can reduce their oxalate content by up to 50%. Therefore, it's important to be aware of how the food is prepared and cooked when assessing its oxalate content.

Consult with a healthcare professional: Consulting with a healthcare professional can help develop a personalized plan to lower oxalate intake, especially if you have a medical condition that makes you more sensitive to oxalates.

Taking supplements: Some supplements like Vitamin B6, Calcium, and magnesium can help lower oxalate levels in the body. Consult with a healthcare professional before taking any supplements.

Chapter 3

Treatment and Management of High Oxalate Levels

Diet and lifestyle changes
Diet and lifestyle changes can be an effective way to manage high oxalate levels and reduce the risk of certain health conditions associated with high oxalate levels.

The most important aspect of diet management is to reduce the intake of oxalate-rich foods such as spinach, beet greens, chocolate, nuts, and certain fruits such as raspberries and blackberries. It is also important to increase the intake of foods that are low in oxalates, such as most fruits and vegetables, meat, fish, and dairy products. Some people may need to follow a strict low-oxalate diet, which is a diet that is specifically designed to minimize the intake of oxalates.

Lifestyle changes that can help manage high oxalate levels include:

- Drinking enough water to help flush out oxalates from the body
- Avoiding foods that can increase the formation of oxalates such as high intake of Vitamin C and calcium supplements
- Avoiding excessive alcohol consumption
- Reducing stress levels

It's also important to work with a healthcare professional, such as a dietitian, who can help create a personalized plan that fits an individual's needs and goals.

It's important to note that reducing oxalate intake alone may not be enough to manage high oxalate levels and it may be necessary to take additional steps such as medications or complementary therapies.

Medications

Medications can be used in addition to diet and lifestyle changes to manage high oxalate levels and reduce the risk of certain health conditions associated with high oxalate levels.

One type of medication that may be used is potassium citrate, which can help to prevent the formation of kidney stones. Potassium citrate works by increasing the pH of urine, making it less acidic and less likely for oxalates to precipitate and form kidney stones.

Another medication that may be used is pyridoxine (vitamin B6), which can help to reduce the formation of oxalates in the body. Studies have shown that pyridoxine can help to lower oxalate levels in the urine, and may be particularly beneficial for people who have a genetic deficiency in the enzyme that metabolizes oxalates.

It's important to note that medications may have side effects and that they should be used under the guidance of a healthcare professional. Medications are not recommended as a first line of treatment, and they should only be used if the diet and lifestyle changes are not enough to manage high oxalate levels.

It's also important to note that while medications may help in managing high oxalate levels, they may not be effective in treating the underlying condition that may have caused the high oxalate levels, such as a metabolic disorder.

Complementary and alternative therapies
Complementary and alternative therapies (CAM) are non-traditional treatments that can be used in addition to diet and lifestyle changes to manage high oxalate levels and

reduce the risk of certain health conditions associated with high oxalate levels.

Some CAM therapies that may help manage high oxalate levels include:

- Chelation therapy: This is a process of removing heavy metals and other toxins from the body through the use of chelating agents such as EDTA. Chelation therapy may help reduce the levels of oxalates in the body, particularly for people with a history of heavy metal exposure.

- Probiotics: Probiotics are live microorganisms that can be taken as supplements to help balance the gut microbiome. Some studies have suggested that probiotics may help to reduce the absorption of oxalates in the gut, which can help to lower oxalate levels in the body.

- Herbal remedies: Some herbal remedies may help to reduce the formation of oxalates in the body, such as chanca piedra and hydrangea root.

It's important to note that CAM therapies should be used under the guidance of a healthcare professional and that they may not be appropriate or effective for everyone. It is important to be aware of the possible side effects and interactions of these therapies with other medications and to check their quality and safety.

It's also important to note that while CAM therapies may help in managing high oxalate levels, they may not be effective in treating the underlying condition that may have caused the high oxalate levels.

- **Working with a healthcare professional**

Working with a healthcare professional is an important aspect of managing high oxalate levels and reducing the risk of certain health conditions associated with high oxalate levels. A healthcare professional can help to identify the underlying cause of high oxalate levels and develop a personalized treatment plan that includes diet and lifestyle changes, medications, and complementary and alternative therapies.

A healthcare professional can help to:

- Diagnose the condition associated with high oxalate levels
- Test for high oxalate levels
- Assess other underlying conditions that may contribute to high oxalate levels
- Guide a low-oxalate diet and other lifestyle changes
- Monitor the effectiveness of treatment
- Guide on taking medications and CAM therapies

It's important to work with a healthcare professional who is familiar with the management of high oxalate levels and related conditions. This may include a nephrologist (kidney specialist), a rheumatologist (arthritis and autoimmune disorder specialist), a neurologist, or a dietitian.

It's important to note that self-diagnosing and self-treating high oxalate levels can be harmful and that a proper diagnosis and treatment plan should be done by a healthcare professional.

Managing Oxalate-Associated Health Conditions

1. Diagnosis and Treatment of Kidney Stones

Diagnosis and treatment of kidney stones associated with high oxalate intake typically involve the following steps:

- **Medical history and physical examination**: A healthcare professional will take a detailed medical history and perform a physical examination to identify any symptoms of kidney stones, such as severe pain in the back, side, or lower abdomen, nausea, and vomiting.

- **Imaging tests:** Imaging tests such as an X-ray, CT scan, or ultrasound can be used to confirm the presence of kidney stones and determine their size and location.

- **Urine tests**: Urine tests can be used to check for the presence of oxalates and other substances that can contribute to the formation of kidney stones.

- **Medical treatment:** The main goal of medical treatment for kidney stones is to relieve pain and prevent complications. Pain medication and anti-nausea medication can be used to relieve pain and vomiting. Drinking plenty of water can also help flush out the kidneys and reduce the formation of crystals.

- **Surgery**: If a kidney stone is too large to pass through the urinary tract, surgery may be necessary to remove it. Surgery may also be necessary if there are complications such as blockages or infections.

- **Diet and lifestyle changes**: Making changes to your diet and lifestyle can help prevent the formation of new kidney stones. This can include avoiding high-oxalate foods, drinking plenty of water, and limiting portion sizes of high-oxalate foods.

- **Medications**: Some medications such as potassium citrate, allopurinol, and sodium cellulose phosphate can be used to prevent the formation of new kidney stones in people with recurrent kidney stones.

It's important to work with a healthcare professional to develop a personalized plan for managing kidney stones associated with high oxalate intake. This may include regular check-ins, imaging tests, and blood tests to monitor the progress of treatment and make adjustments as needed.

2. **Managing Autoimmune Disease:** Managing autoimmune disease associated with high oxalate intake typically involves the following steps:

Medical history and physical examination: A healthcare professional will take a detailed medical history and perform a physical examination to identify any symptoms of autoimmune disease such as joint pain, fatigue, and skin rashes.

Laboratory tests: Blood tests, such as the ANA (antinuclear antibody) test, ESR (erythrocyte sedimentation rate) and CRP (C-reactive protein) test can be used to diagnose autoimmune disease and to monitor the progress of treatment.

Medical treatment: The main goal of medical treatment for autoimmune diseases is to reduce inflammation and prevent damage to the body's tissues. This may include the use of non-steroidal anti-inflammatory drugs (NSAIDs), corticosteroids, and disease-modifying antirheumatic drugs (DMARDs).

Diet and lifestyle changes: Making changes to your diet and lifestyle can help reduce inflammation and prevent the progression of autoimmune disease. This can include avoiding high oxalate foods, consuming low oxalate foods, and consuming a diet rich in fruits and vegetables.

Physical therapy and exercise: Physical therapy and exercise can help reduce pain and improve mobility in people with autoimmune diseases.

Medications: Some medications such as biological drugs (like TNF inhibitors) can be used to treat autoimmune disease, these medications can be used in combination with the above strategies.

It's important to be aware of the potential triggers for autoimmune diseases, such as stress, infection, and environmental toxins, and to take steps to avoid or manage them. Additionally, some people may benefit from complementary therapies such as acupuncture, massage therapy, and yoga to help manage symptoms.

It's important to note that autoimmune disease is complex, and there is no one-size-fits-all approach to management. It may take time and experimentation to find the right combination of treatments that work for you. It's also important to be patient and consistent with the treatment plan, as it can take time to see improvement.

3. **Managing Neurological and Gastrointestinal Symptoms**: Managing neurological and gastrointestinal symptoms associated with high oxalate intake typically involves the following steps:

   - **Medical history and physical examination**: A healthcare professional will take a detailed medical history and perform a physical examination to identify any symptoms such as neuropathy, seizures, abdominal pain, diarrhea, and constipation.

- **Diagnostic tests:** Tests such as nerve conduction studies, MRI scans and colonoscopy may be done to confirm the presence of neurological or gastrointestinal symptoms and identify any underlying causes.

- **Medical treatment:** The main goal of medical treatment for neurological and gastrointestinal symptoms is to relieve pain and prevent complications. Medications can be used to relieve pain, control seizures, and manage diarrhea and constipation.

- **Diet and lifestyle changes:** Making changes to your diet and lifestyle can help reduce symptoms and prevent the progression of neurological and gastrointestinal symptoms. This can include avoiding high-oxalate foods, consuming low-oxalate foods, and drinking plenty of water.

- **Physical therapy and exercise**: Physical therapy and exercise can help reduce pain and improve mobility in people with neurological symptoms.

- **Medications**: Some medications such as anticonvulsants and antidepressants may be used to manage neurological symptoms, and medications such as laxatives and antispasmodics may be used to manage gastrointestinal symptoms.

- **Complementary therapies:** Some people may benefit from complementary therapies such as acupuncture, massage therapy, and yoga to help manage symptoms.

It's important to work with a healthcare professional to develop a personalized plan for managing neurological and gastrointestinal symptoms associated with high oxalate intake, monitoring the progress of treatment, and making adjustments as needed.

Conclusion

Summary of Key Points

In conclusion, oxalates are naturally occurring compounds found in many foods and play a role in the body, but high oxalate intake can lead to various health conditions such as kidney stones, autoimmune disease, and neurological and gastrointestinal symptoms.

Identifying high oxalate foods is important in managing oxalate intake and reducing the risk of harm, using a combination of laboratory testing, food databases, consulting a dietitian or healthcare professional, and home testing kits.

Lowering oxalate intake can be achieved by avoiding high oxalate foods, limiting portion sizes of high oxalate foods, drinking plenty of water, cooking and preparation methods, consulting with a healthcare professional, and taking supplements.

Managing health conditions associated with high oxalate intakes such as kidney stones, autoimmune disease, and neurological and gastrointestinal symptoms involves a combination of medical treatment, diet and lifestyle changes, physical therapy and exercise, and medications.

It's important to work with a healthcare professional to develop a personalized plan for managing these health conditions, monitoring the progress of treatment, and making adjustments as needed.

It is important to note that everyone's dietary needs and sensitivities are different and that what might be a high-oxalate food for one person may not be for another.

Additionally, some people may need to follow a low-oxalate diet to manage certain health conditions, such as kidney stones or primary hyperoxaluria. In these cases, it's essential to work with a healthcare professional to create a personalized diet plan that works for you.

Future research on oxalates should focus on a few key areas, including:

1. Understanding the underlying causes of high oxalate levels: While it is known that certain foods and genetic factors can contribute to high oxalate levels, more research is needed to fully understand the underlying causes of this condition.

2. Investigating the link between oxalates and various health conditions: While some studies have suggested that high oxalate levels may be associated with certain health conditions, more research is needed to confirm these associations and to

understand the underlying mechanisms.

3. Developing new treatments: While diet and lifestyle changes, medications, and complementary and alternative therapies can help to manage high oxalate levels, more research is needed to develop new and more effective treatments for this condition.

4. Examining the impact of oxalates in a different population: More research is needed to understand how oxalates affect different population groups such as children, the elderly, and people with comorbidities.

5. Investigating the role of oxalates in gut health: Oxalates can affect gut health and the gut microbiome, future research should investigate the role of

oxalates in gut health and how it can affect overall health.

Resources for Further Information

There are several resources available for further information on oxalates and high oxalate levels. These include:

1. National Kidney Foundation: The National Kidney Foundation is a leading organization in kidney health and provides information on the prevention, diagnosis, and treatment of kidney stones, including information on oxalates.

2. The Oxford Stone Group: The Oxford Stone Group is a research group dedicated to understanding the causes and management of kidney stones, and provides information on oxalate metabolism and the dietary management of kidney stones.

3. The Low Oxalate Diet Support Group: This is a support group for individuals who are following a low oxalate diet and provides information and support for people who are managing high oxalate levels.

4. The Fibromyalgia and Chronic Fatigue Center: This center provides information and resources on fibromyalgia and chronic fatigue syndrome, including information on the role of oxalates in these conditions.

5. International Society for Autism Research: This society provides information on the latest research and developments in autism research, including information on the role of oxalates in autism.

It's important to note that information found online should be critically evaluated, and it's recommended to consult a healthcare professional before making any changes to your diet or lifestyle.

Printed in Great Britain
by Amazon